G :

# WITH YOUR
## BETTER MENTAL HEALTH

A guide to managing anxiety, one of humanity's biggest challenges

GET IN TOUCH SERIES



Michael Terence Publishing

First published in paperback by
Michael Terence Publishing in 2021
www.mtp.agency



ISBN 9781800941755



Cover designed by Glow Designs
www.glow-designs.co.uk

# CONTENTS

INTRODUCTION ........................................................ 1

THE SOURCE OF ANXIETY ........................................ 3

THE THREE TYPES OF ANXIETY .................................. 6

PRIMARY AND SECONDARY ANXIETIES .................... 10

THE PARENT OF ALL ANXIETY: UNCERTAINTY ......... 14

ANXIETY AND SHOCK ............................................. 18

ANXIETY AND ADDICTIONS .................................... 21

ANXIETY AND THE MEDIA ...................................... 25

ANXIETY AND DIGITAL ADDICTION ......................... 29

ANXIETY AND TECHNOLOGY BURNOUT .................. 33

ANXIETY AND INSOMNIA ....................................... 36

ANXIETY AND LONELINESS ..................................... 41

ANXIETY AND FEAR ................................................ 44

ANXIETY AND PHOBIAS .......................................... 48

THE BRAIN-GUT PARADOX ..................................... 54

DIAGNOSTIC LABELLING AND SECONDARY GAIN .. 58

MANAGING A DIAGNOSIS....................................................63
EPIGENETIC AND INHERITED ANXIETY .....................66
OBSESSIVE COMPULSIVE DISORDER ........................70
TRADITIONAL VERSUS ALTERNATIVE THERAPY .......74
HYPNOSIS......................................................................79
MEDITATION ...............................................................83
EXERCISE......................................................................87
NATURE AND ANIMALS..............................................92
HUMOUR.......................................................................96

CONCLUSION ...............................................................99

ALSO IN THE GET IN TOUCH SERIES ..................... 101

# INTRODUCTION

*'Nothing is permanent in this wicked world.*
*Not even our troubles.'*

– Charlie Chaplin

It's an interesting thought, but if your ancestors hadn't been anxious you wouldn't be around to read this book. Why is that? We will go into much more depth about this, but in the first instance it is because our ancestors lived with very different anxieties, ones which they were perfectly adapted to deal with. Genetically we have inherited those life-saving anxieties, but, in the twenty-first century, we do not have to deal with tigers in the jungle whilst hunting for our dinner. Our brains don't know this, however, and are responsible for sending us into the same flight, fight or freeze response to modern-day anxieties in the form of overwork, stress, financial worries, economic changes – the list for everyone is different – that we needed when faced with the tiger in the long grass.

Before we continue, I'd like to share with you the reason for writing this book. I have a history of acute and chronic anxiety, which I worked on for years to the point of successful management on a daily basis. My quest for a solution led me to pursue a career in nursing care with the NHS, where I trained in psychotherapy at Regents College, London. After qualifying, I worked closely with doctors at my local surgery in London, and as a private practitioner from home. I am currently still caring for my one hundred-year-old father, who lives at home with me. Therefore, this book has been written by someone who knows how it feels to be completely overcome by anxiety, but who knows first-hand that it is possible to learn to manage this life-threatening state. I hope you benefit from what I have written, and please pass this book on to anyone who you think might need it too.

Anxiety is one of the biggest challenges to mental and physical health humanity has had to face. This book is a discussion of the sources of general anxiety, and more personal anxieties too. I feel confident I have covered many of the causes and symptoms of anxiety and, more importantly, have offered simple, practical exercises to help you deal with your modern-day tigers.

# THE SOURCE OF ANXIETY

*'Anxiety does not empty tomorrow of its sorrows, but only empties today of its strength.'*
– Charles Spurgeon

Where does anxiety and worry come from? It is vitally important to understand the source of all anxiety, as only then will you start to conquer it.

Interestingly, anxiety is your friend and without it you wouldn't get far. All living organisms have one thing in common and that is to survive. There is nothing more fundamental to any organism than this fact. Everything, from a virus to a mammal, spends their whole existence trying to survive, but the big difference between us and every other organism on the planet is that we get anxious about survival, they don't.

All living systems want to continue their species and will reproduce, adapt and mutate to give them the best chance of generational longevity. To survive as one of the lowest lifeforms is purely mechanistic. In higher lifeforms it becomes instinctive, and in humans it developed into rational thinking. The element of the brain known as the reptilian brain, or the brainstem (primal brain), goes back one hundred million years. This part of the brain is in charge of anxiety, which is a physical response to danger. The limbic system controls emotions which refer to anxiety; and the neocortex, or the rational brain, causes anxiety, which becomes relevant in rational thinking humans.

The fundamental cause of extreme, unrelenting anxiety is an internal conflict between different elements of the brain and the body. When one aspect of the organism is out of sync with others, crippling anxiety occurs, because the brain is unable to recognise that the anxiety – the initial event or threat that may have triggered the physical response – has passed, and keeps playing it over and over again, thus reaffirming that there is still a threat of some kind around when, in actual fact, it's just the recollection of the threat.

This loop is highly destructive, and we must learn to recognise it, because despite anxiety serving a purpose in that it can protect us, unprocessed anxiety that is allowed to keep playing out in the brain will make us mentally and physically ill. But you know this, I'm sure, which is why you are reading this book.

## THINGS TO TRY

Anxiety has a purpose, but make friends with your brain rather than giving it a hard time. Recognise the anxiety, and thank your brain for bringing a threat to your attention. But when the threat has passed, or if it is just a replay of an old threat, tell your brain it's okay now. This may sound too simple, but it is something we will discuss a lot, and an exercise you will grow to love.

# THE THREE TYPES OF ANXIETY

*'Behind every flinch is a fear or an anxiety, sometimes rational, sometimes not.'*

– Julien Smith

Anxiety can be split into three levels: **irrational anxiety; semi-irrational anxiety; rational anxiety.**

**Irrational anxiety** is defined as worry that is completely without reason. Fear of falling off the moon would be defined as an irrational anxiety.

**Semi-irrational anxiety** comes under the banner of the 'What if?' syndrome. In other words, there is a possibility of something happening, even though it is very unlikely. For example, it is possible that one might die of a rare disease or be killed in a future war, but what are the chances? This type of anxiety emerges from the remote possibility of something happening, and the very thought of it is enough to set an anxious brain into a tailspin. In my experience as a psychotherapist, the What if? syndrome seems to love a slightly hyperactive, analytic brain, and can create all manner of possibilities: What if I got run over by a bus tomorrow? banged my head and lost my memory? lost my job because I couldn't remember how to do it? couldn't pay my mortgage because I was unemployable? On and on and on... Equally, it can affect just about anybody who overthinks a thing to the point of it taking over.

Superstition is another version of semi-irrational anxiety. We've all heard people say that walking under a ladder will bring bad luck – most likely because someone, once, a very long time ago, walked under a ladder and then maybe crossed the road and got hit by a bus...! The brain prone to semi-irrational anxiety loves this kind of thing, and the false fear of bad luck being the result of walking under a ladder is triggered by the very sight of the ladder, never mind the act of walking under it, and will wander off into all sorts of possible scenarios, the chances of which are highly remote. As a result, the superstition feeds the anxiety, and the anxiety makes sure you continue to believe the superstition.

**Rational anxiety** is a very 'real-time' anxiety. Worrying about failing an exam if you haven't studied enough, or messing up a speaking event because you haven't practised enough, or getting a disease because you smoke one hundred cigarettes a day are all examples of 'real' anxiety. In an extreme case, someone pointing a loaded gun at you is a very real cause of anxiety.

However, much of our anxiety is irrational or semi-irrational, and we spend most of our lives worrying about things that simply won't happen – or are extremely unlikely to happen. Here is an example:

I once attended a lecture by a psychologist who described how he gave a motivational talk to a group of pensioners. He proceeded to enquire as to the thing they feared most. Their answer? Going out at night. He followed this up by asking 'Why are you afraid of going out?' Most responded the same way: Because of the fear of being attacked.

Our speaker then explained that the most risky place for the retired population was, in actual fact, their own home, because we are far more likely to suffer an injury around the house than taking a stroll in the evening and being attacked by a stranger. He obviously wasn't trying to make them afraid of their own homes, but rather bring to their attention the huge gulf between the *fear* of being attacked and the *possibility* of it actually happening.

So why do we develop all sorts of irrational fears and anxieties? In essence, we use them as a security blanket to keep us from the remote chance of danger, a buffer against the dangerous world 'out there' and our perceived safety 'in here'. But this is not healthy, we all know that. Try this exercise and see how you feel after a few weeks.

## THINGS TO TRY

Is your anxiety irrational, semi-irrational, or rational? Write it down, or write them all down. Look at them. Analyse them. This will help you to separate them into real and not real. The ones that are real...tell the brain they're made up, it will start to listen soon enough. The real ones...these you can do something about: study harder, practice that speech, cut down or, better still, give up smoking. This gives YOU the power over your anxieties and fears, not the other way around.

# PRIMARY AND SECONDARY ANXIETIES

*'Be aware of your breathing as often as you are able, whenever you remember. And it's free.'*
– Eckhart Tolle

Anxiety is split into two groups: **survival anxieties** and **secondary anxieties.**

**Survival anxieties** can include fear of death, fears around relationships and/or the inability to procreate, fear of not being accepted, and fear of uncertainty. (Later in the book we will break these fears down to several elements, including survival verses non-survival addictions.)

**Secondary anxieties** can include fear of pain, disease, loneliness, failure, being laughed at, or social interactions. They can trigger obsessive compulsive disorders (OCDs), phobias, social anxiety, superstitions, guilt complexes and various elements of neurosis.

Interestingly, survival anxiety is fundamental to human existence, and in its purest, most primitive form invariably meant the difference between life or death: separation or not being accepted by our tribe or clan was a serious life threat. When our survival is threatened at this level our physiology is directly affected, driven by a part of the brain called the amygdala, which results in increased adrenaline, increased heartrate, shallow, rapid breathing, sweating, and an interruption to the digestive system. These **sympathetic** physiological responses prepare the body for action, often called the fight, flight or freeze response. When the threat passes, the **parasympathetic** responses kick in, which bring the body back to its normal state.

Fears about survival, or because of a secondary issue like fear of social interactions, become a problem for humans when we are unable to turn off the fight, flight or freeze response. The adrenaline keeps pumping, the heart keeps pounding, and suddenly we are in the throes of an anxiety or panic attack. You know that feeling? So how can we treat these causes of crippling anxiety, not just when they occur, but in the longer term?

In the immediate moment, we must force ourselves to **breathe**. In the longer term, there are many ways to address the deeper, underlying causes of the anxiety, many of which we will go on to discuss.

## THINGS TO TRY

This breathing exercise can be practised at any time of the day, not just when we are in a state of anxiety or panic. In fact, the more you make it a habit to spend time focussing on your breathing when you are calm, the easier it will be to apply the practice when you become anxious.

This practice is called **abdominal breathing**, and it works like this:

Breathe in from the abdomen, or stomach, quite literally pushing it out whilst you inhale. Count to four as you inhale, and hold the breath for a count of four. Then exhale for a count of four, allowing the abdomen to retract. Do this several times. You will feel your heartrate naturally slow whether you are anxious or not. Some people find it advantageous to place their hand on their abdomen to ensure that it is moving rather than their upper chest.

When you become comfortable doing this, begin to lengthen the exhale for a count of six or eight. (I sometimes find it helps to yawn on the exhale, as it increases the effect of the out breath.)

Do this several times during the day. You can do it sitting at your desk, watching TV, reading a book, it doesn't matter. But make sure you relax into the practice and do not force it. Enjoy it. Feel your heartrate slowing and your body thanking you for the extra oxygen.

If you find yourself in a situation where you feel the anxiety rising, or even if it has beat you to it and already has, remember to breathe like this. It only takes a few breaths to start the body's calming, parasympathetic process.

In extreme cases, breathing in and out of a paper bag for no more than half a minute can reset the carbon dioxide and oxygen imbalance caused by overwhelming anxiety. Abdominal breathing requires nothing more than your focus, so keep practising. Try it right now, if you like?

# THE PARENT OF ALL ANXIETY: UNCERTAINTY

*'Present fears are less than horrible imaginings.'*
– William Shakespeare

Many people find uncertainty almost unbearable. We are creatures of habit in the present, but we also like to plan our future based on those habits, or certainties. When certainty is removed, for instance if we lose our job or our relationship ends, we can often find ourselves in a state of mild or even intense panic.

Let's take Covid-19 as a very current example. We are swamped with uncertainties. It is not certain whether will get the virus or not. It is not certain whether someone you encounter in the supermarket or petrol station might have it. Some of us are uncertain about future employment and travel. We are uncertain about the vaccine, and whether to have it or not. We are uncertain when we will next see our relatives and friends. We are uncertain whether to believe everything (or anything at all) that comes out of our

TV screens... If there is anything that creates anxiety it is uncertainty.

Uncertainty is closely linked to expectation. When we fall in love we have a high expectation of happiness and security. Until we fall in love, we might be anxious about ever finding a partner. And when we do, the act of being in love is desirable, primarily because it reduces uncertainty. If the relationship looks like it might go wrong uncertainty returns, and often we face the dilemma of trying to make an unhappy relationship work just to quell that uncertainty. There is much expectation and reliance on spiritual and religious beliefs for the same reason, largely because we are uncertain what happens to us when we die. We derive comfort from our beliefs as they give us something to hold on to, despite there often being a certain amount of uncertainty as to whether they are true or not.

We desperately look for certainty in our lives, because uncertainty often requires making choices that create even more anxiety than the uncertainty itself! What if I make the wrong choice? Shall I leave him/her or not? Shall I believe what the sage or vicar tells me or not? (The paradox, oddly enough, is that once a choice has been made it actually lessens the anxiety.)

People who suffer from both survival and secondary anxiety are the most prone to uncertainty anxiety, and often when one fear is resolved it is immediately replaced by another. Try this exercise, which is used by the military.

## THINGS TO TRY

To cope with uncertainty anxiety you need to benchmark certain rituals in your day which help to calm the brain and convince it all is well. The military use benchmark rituals to help prepare men and women for war.

When you get up in the morning have a regular sequence of events that you always stick to. They don't require any skill or thought, but act as an ordered feedback to your psyche. They can include things like making your bed, cleaning your teeth, going for a walk, meditating, reading, stretching – whatever you like to do. The options are endless, but they must be carried out on a daily basis.

Uncertainty is a fact of life and cannot be avoided. Morning rituals create order, both psychologically and literally, and make us better able to cope with the anxiety triggered by uncertainty.

# ANXIETY AND SHOCK

*'Smile, breathe, and go slowly.'*

– Thich Nhat Hanh

Shock is the result of acute anxiety, usually following a physical trauma of some kind, like excessive cold or heat, dehydration, exhaustion, injury or accident.

Shock can also be triggered by traumatic psychological events, such as sudden bad news, verbal or physical aggression, combat, or an unexpected sight like the discovery of a dead body.

Shock is technically a medical condition. It is defined as a reduction of circulating fluid (mainly blood) to the vital organs. These vital organs consist of the heart, brain, kidneys, liver, lungs, spleen etc., which are the systems that control all the functions of the body. Shock is also connected to the vagus nervous system, which connects these organs and sends messages between the brain and the body, and will cause similar symptoms to that of medical shock.

People in shock look pale and their skin will be clammy. The heartrate increases, and their breathing becomes rapid and shallow. They may feel sick, or vomit, and appear vacant. These symptoms are the result of the body trying to deal with the shock in an attempt to send more blood to the vital organs. This balancing process is known as homeostasis.

The anxiety associated with shock in most instances lessens as soon as the body begins to recover physically. Psychologically the shock may linger, however, and this is when shock anxiety might become apparent. There is lots of information online about this, and how to manage it, but here is a simple exercise which will help.

## THINGS TO TRY

If you know your anxiety is linked to a physical or psychological shock you may have had, and the physical symptoms of shock keep returning as if you are right back there, it's because your brain has not been able to separate the past event from the present, where the shock has passed. Recognising this is the first step to managing post-shock anxiety.

The brain is a powerful tool, but it only believes what it is told. When the symptoms and the anxiety return, remind the brain that the shock was in the past, and redirect the strong, negative energy of the memory into a strong, positive action, like reminding yourself how lucky you are to be safe now. A body and brain in shock only wants to get home, where it is safe. This 'safe now' message, when combined with abdominal breathing if you need to, is deeply calming. Practise this, and in time the brain will process the shock and remember all is now well.

# ANXIETY AND ADDICTIONS

*'Anxiety is the handmaiden of creativity.'*

– T.S. Elliot

There are two addictions that directly relate to primary survival anxiety, and they are **overeating** and **sexual addictions** in all their forms.

Conditions like obsessive compulsive disorder and anorexia are more related to secondary anxiety, and are used to maintain some form of control over the anxiety. We will be talking about these more shortly, but first let's look at the addictions triggered by survival anxieties.

Our ancestors never knew when the next meal was coming, so to survive they needed to pack away as many fats, sugars and carbohydrates as possible. Consequently, they gorged on whatever was available to gain the weight which would keep them going during the lean times.

When we become anxious on a primary, survival level, the brain is tricked into thinking our survival is at risk and therefore it craves fattening foods to keep us going. Carbohydrates also have the added advantage of improving the levels of the neurotransmitter serotonin in the brain, which makes us feel happy. (Perhaps why many people feel more depressed in the morning, and if their blood sugar level drops during the day.) Comfort eating is a real thing, not just an expression, and survival-anxious people become addicted to food as their comforter.

Sexual addiction has a similar effect in people crippled by survival anxiety. The anxiety convinces the brain that it is in danger, creating the desire to procreate. (This phenomenon also has the effect of making partners more fertile when in starvation mode.) Sexual arousal floods the brain with dopamine, which can cause an addictive reaction and make people more promiscuous. If they can't find an outlet, they may resort to pornography.

Secondary anxieties will lead to other addictions. Alcohol and narcotic drugs are used to both to create courage – if the secondary anxiety is social interaction, for instance – and dull the associated anxiety. They trick the brain into thinking all is well...but the effect never lasts.

Addictions like OCD and anorexia can also be the result of secondary anxieties, like loneliness or fear of failure. We might develop a deep anxiety about catching a disease, and think that if we say a certain word one hundred times as we walk down the street, or only walk down the left-hand side of the street, we will be safe. A young girl or boy may feel lonely at school, and feel they have no control over who likes them or not, so starving themselves puts them in control of their lives. This control over everything we eat, or obsessive repetition of words, also tricks the brain into thinking all is well...but the effect never lasts, and sometimes the addictive behaviour becomes more and more extreme to counter the further anxiety.

Not all anxious people develop addictions, but this exercise might help if you have.

**THINGS TO TRY**

Replacement addictions are very powerful, and are designed to get you addicted to something that will benefit you in some way.

At the core of every anxious, addicted human is the voice that says there is another way. For instance, chewing gum can trick the brain into thinking it has eaten, and help avoid the addiction to eating. Another way, and better for us, is to do something active when the anxiety and urge to eat kicks in, like go for a walk, or dance to some loud music. The brain is lazy though, and it wants to give in, so we may have to be quite forceful to begin with to help it become addicted to something new.

Sexual addictions can be replaced with creativity, like writing or painting, which triggers dopamine in the brain. Getting involved in something productive, like volunteering at the local hospice, also replaces the addiction with something positive and reminds us that we are not alone.

If you really are struggling, there are several organisations that use group therapy to deal with addictions, like Alcoholics Anonymous, which now has many other groups for all sorts of other addictions.

# ANXIETY AND THE MEDIA

*'Nothing is worth poisoning yourself into stress, anxiety, and fear.'*

– Steve Maraboli

Cravings are dictated by physical dependency, whereas habits are dictated by emotional dependency.

There is no doubt that anxiety can mean the development of bad habits. Physical dependency on cravings, or bad habits, is the result of chemicals released in the brain. But bad habits cause further anxiety, which leads to further dependency. The media is one such 'bad habit' and can manipulate your brain through habitual conscious and subconscious abuse.

There are two types of media that influence our brains. The first is **traditional media**, where information is fed with little or no interaction from the viewer or listener. The second is **social media,** where the viewer can interact with the source with almost no accountability. Both types of media can be highly negative and extremely toxic. If so, why is negative media so popular?

As discussed, we are hardwired to survive and are always on the lookout for danger. When we hear or see something negative on the news or read it in a paper, we pay attention, as we might be at risk. The media moguls know this, and therefore feed us more of the same, knowing we will become hooked to every latest bulletin and update. They also know we are willing to pay for this news through our subscriptions to various newspapers and twenty-four-hour-a-day streamed TV channels. Few people know that the continuous feeding of this stuff affects our brain, causing neurotic thinking and anxiety.

When it comes to social media, the affect is exactly the same, except that we can participate from our phones and other devices, thus feeding the negativity and increasing the toxic effects of bad news – both for ourselves and others. Data reveals that most people reach for their phones within five minutes of waking, and spend anything from ten minutes to an hour or more during this crucial time of day for the waking brain feeding it negative news. We might then get up and put the TV on, and have more negative news playing away in the background as we begin our day. And we wonder why we are anxious...

**It is my absolute belief that if we avoided media and social media a great deal of our anxiety would dissipate.**

Unfortunately, the extreme negativity of both these media sources directly affect our brains, releasing the chemicals that mean we crave more of the same. And what started out as curiosity about a news item becomes an addiction that feeds our anxiety, and soon has us imagining all manner of other horrors and scenarios, that feed straight back to the anxiety. **We have to break this cycle if we are to tackle our anxiety.**

## THINGS TO TRY

Seriously limit your exposure to media and social media. Have a catch-up once a day if you really need to, but then turn the TV off or put your phone down. And definitely avoid watching or reading just before bed and the moment you wake up. Endless commentary on the day's issues feeds anxiety. Give your brain half a chance and feed it something positive instead, like some great music or an interesting, uplifting podcast.

Whilst social media can keep us company, it is now known that it is addictive due to high levels of chemicals released in the brain. Again, have a news catch-up once a day if you need to, and then choose to read something that is uplifting, powerful and makes you feel good. And definitely do not get involved in toxic, negative discussions that feed not just your anxiety but others' too. Your amazing brain deserves better, so give it something to read it will thank you for.

# ANXIETY AND DIGITAL ADDICTION

*'The opposite of addiction is human connection.'*
– Johann Hari

Why can becoming addicted to our phones and devices be so harmful? And why does it cause such anxiety?

Digital addiction is triggered by a two things. Firstly, there is the drive for validation; a desire for recognition which can develop into anxiety, depression and narcissism. Like all drugs - and the dopamine high in the brain caused by checking our phones is very addictive - the hit becomes less effective as time passes, and we need even more validation. At one time twenty 'Likes' might have been enough, but soon you crave more. When you get fifty Likes, you want a hundred, etc... And when the Likes start decreasing, or you start losing friends or followers, this can cause deep anxiety and even depression.

The second trigger is what I call the 'link addiction', or the dopamine high just before you press the next link, and the next link, taking you deeper into an online world and away from the real world around you. This detaches you from your surroundings, and can make it very hard to relate to the actual people and situations around you, which can also cause great anxiety, loneliness and depression.

We have all seen really young children in their pushchairs or in the supermarket trolley with a phone or other device propped up in front of them to 'keep them quiet', much the same as a dummy is used with babies. Is it any wonder that addiction to technology has become what it is? It has been triggered at this early age, when children could be interacting with the people around them or learning about the different foods in the supermarket. As more and more children have their own smart phone or tablet, the more this addiction will increase. It is not helped, in my opinion, by using tablets in schools instead of books. Young brains, although ostensibly learning, are becoming addicted to screens. Often when they are not in front of a screen they have no idea what to do with themselves, and become anxious and disruptive as they crave the high from looking at their devices. In a similar way, as teenagers and adults we simply do not seem to be able to break our addiction to our phones. So what can we do?

## THINGS TO TRY

Become your own screen-time manager and quite literally book time off and time on your devices. Aside from work-related screen-time, allow yourself half an hour in the morning, at lunchtime, and maybe an hour in the evening. That is still *two hours* a day spent on your phone. What else could you do with that time?

Force yourself – and your children – to enjoy some offline activities like going to the park or chucking a ball about in the garden. Anything to get you away from your phones and into each other's company.

If you have to spend a lot of time on your phone or computer because of work or study, book yourself some screen-breaks – and *real* breaks. Go into a different room, away from your phone and computer, and do something completely different, like bake a cake or mow the lawn or do some exercise. Again, anything to get you away from your devices.

Look at the screen-time record on your phone and work out how much of that time was not work-related. I think you will be shocked. We must break this addiction by filling the time with events that bond us to the humans in our lives. A screen cannot put its arm around you when you become anxious and depressed.

# ANXIETY AND TECHNOLOGY BURNOUT

*'Almost everything will work again if you unplug for a few minutes, including you.'*

– Anne Lamott

The use of digital technology, particularly recently, has almost reached saturation point. How many more hours a day can we spend in front of a screen of some kind working, doing research, studying, having meetings, conducting counselling sessions – the list goes on and on – without suffering from technology burnout? What can be an addiction, as discussed in the previous chapter, can also become the source of overwhelming anxiety and exhaustion, something which the health community are ill-equipped to deal with. How do you treat screen anxiety?

The anxiety associated with technology can be split into three. Firstly, there is the technological side itself, and perhaps the anxiety it will fail us in the middle of a meeting or counselling session – and this applies equally to those on both sides of the meeting or session. Secondly, there is the overwhelming amount of advice on every subject known to man, which can be exhausting when trying to do research for work or an assignment. Thirdly, there is the lack of normal stimulus online that helps us navigate a meeting or counselling session and gauge how best to respond, which works two ways: we're unsure of the authenticity of the reactions we might get on a screen; and we wonder if we are coming across as authentic, which can cause a lack of confidence and much anxiety.

So how can we combat screen anxiety, and feel relaxed and confident and not overwhelmed by the effect of being on our computer for so long?

## THINGS TO TRY

With respect to the first point, there are certain things we can do to ensure our technology doesn't fail, like make sure we have enough battery time or we're plugged in, or make sure our broadband isn't overloaded during the meeting by people streaming in another room. But nothing is failsafe, and remembering we all have the same issues with technology and mentioning it at the beginning of the meeting or counselling session goes a long way in calming the anxiety.

When it comes to the amount of advice online on any given subject, don't be tempted to keep clicking link after link, which can often take us away from the specific subject we need to research. Stick to well-reputed sources, and a small selection.

At the start of meetings or sessions, put the other parties at ease by mentioning that online communication can sometimes be hard, and that you will do your best to be clear in your speech. Ask the other parties to tell you if you are unclear, and don't be afraid to ask someone to repeat themselves if you haven't quite understood their point. Anything we can do to make our online encounters as relaxed as possible helps us and the person/people we are talking to less anxious.

# ANXIETY AND INSOMNIA

*'Oh Soul. You worry too much.
You have seen your own strength.'*

– Rumi

We all need sleep to process the day's activities and rest our body. Dreaming is a big part of that processing. But what can we do when anxiety keeps us awake? Worse, worrying about not being able to sleep makes the anxiety worse, which is known as an anxiety loop: the more you worry the more you worry about worrying. Further to this, if you invest a lot of time worrying, your subconscious assumes there is something to worry about, and feeds back the need to worry more.

The majority of adults need around seven to eight hours sleep in a twenty-four hour period, but we all have different sleep pattens and sleep doesn't necessarily have to be all at one time. During primitive life, sleep naturally occurred at night as the day was for working the land. Modern life is very different, with many of us working night shifts, or much later into the night out of choice, and, although not ideal, if you are able to sleep in sections throughout the day this is still OK. Whenever you do go to sleep, however, it's important to make your room as dark as possible, covering the windows to simulate night-time.

There is so much information out there about creating good sleeping habits. We teach our children to do this, getting them into a routine of a warm bath, a warm drink, and maybe reading them a story before bed. So why is it as adults that we often stop doing this, watching loud, bright TV until late at night, or spending hours glued to our phones and other devices? Often we snack on salty or sugary foods too, and drink too much caffeine or alcohol, none of which induce a good night's sleep. These stimulants play havoc in our bloodstream, and the combination of this and having a mind prone to worrying is not a good combination. We also work far too late, sending last-minute emails about work or over-stimulating our minds by suddenly debating a work issue in our heads.

Anything we can do to prepare the mind and body for sleep will help to ease anxiety, becoming a habit that the subconscious latches onto as the thought: *Ah, now it's time to sleep*. We are all different in our habits, but here are some exercises that are well worth trying until you find something that works for you.

## THINGS TO TRY

The body's temperature drops when we are tired, which naturally prepares us for a warm bed and sleep. Try getting into bed slightly cold and allowing the bed to warm you up. Often this simple thing helps you to drift off to sleep.

Try not to eat late at night, instead enjoying a good meal earlier in the evening. And definitely avoid tea, coffee or alcohol late at night. Have a soothing drink instead, like a herbal tea or warm, milky drink.

Stay away from negative media and social media for at least two hours before bed and avoid going to sleep with the TV on. Quiet, relaxing music playing in the background instead might help you drift off, but avoid anything that is too stirring or triggers memories that might trigger anxiety.

During my very anxious times I would use a repetitive thought process before bed, rather like the old sheep-counting method. As a great lover of squash in my younger days, I would imagine hitting the ball slowly to the back wall over and over again. Rehearsing a non-anxious repetitive activity like this really works. (It also improved my squash!) Similarly, if you have a goal or desire night time is a good time to meditate on it, but using the repetition of a single phrase or thought rather than mulling over a thousand ideas which will over-stimulate the brain.

Make sure your bed is comfortable and the pillows are just right for you. It's amazing the difference the right pillow can make, and again signals to the brain that it's now time to sleep.

Certain aromatic smells can also help. Visit your local health shop for advice.

Gentle stretching can ease out the tensions of the day, relaxing the muscles and the mind. But nothing too strenuous. The point is to prompt relaxation not stimulation. Repeating a phrase or thought, as above, as you do this again helps to prepare the body and brain for sleep.

If insomnia is becoming a serious problem you might consider getting some help. The anxiety-insomnia-anxiety loop is awful, so please don't be afraid to talk to your GP. There may be other underlying factors, like snoring or sleep apnoea, that they can help you with. Anything you do to undo the anxiety loop is a positive message to your subconscious as you approach bedtime.

# ANXIETY AND LONELINESS

*'There are far, far better things ahead than anything we leave behind.'*

– C.S. Lewis

I wouldn't say that loneliness actually causes anxiety, but it can magnify it. We are designed to be part of a community, the most natural being the family unit. Research has shown, however, that it is the quality of relationships that provides the biggest protection against loneliness, so if we struggle to identify with family, or don't have a close family, we can create a surrogate family in good friends.

Loneliness can arise for a number of reasons, like the death of a life partner, or moving to a new place, and we must find ways to connect with people if we find ourselves getting anxious, as the anxiety can sometimes make the loneliness feel more acute. Joining coffee mornings or clubs with shared interests can quickly put us in touch with potential friends, as can signing up for community projects or attending a local church.

As a society we can all play our part in helping our fellow humans to find each other, not just because we might be a little lonely but because others might be lonely too. People are often ashamed to admit they are lonely, so take the initiative. Doing so, ironically, may make us a little anxious to begin with, as meeting new people doesn't come naturally to some of us; but when we do, and find ourselves laughing over shared experiences or connecting through an art club or singing group, the anxiety is soon replaced by the joy of that connection.

## THINGS TO TRY

Visit your local library or look online to see what clubs and groups are in your area. You might want to join a club you are familiar with, or even try something you've never done before. Both will put you in touch with people who may fill the gap loneliness can create.

Thinking about other people and their possible loneliness – like the elderly, for instance – takes the focus off our own feelings and helps us to connect with those of others.

In the UK also has programmes like 'social prescribing' where health professionals refer patients to communities and groups which can help with health and general wellbeing. Joining communities like these really does help to reduce loneliness and, as a consequence, the anxiety that may come with it.

# ANXIETY AND FEAR

*'Do not anticipate trouble or worry about what may never happen. Keep in the sunlight.'*

– Benjamin Franklin

In the chapter on the three types of anxiety, irrational anxiety, once recognised, can be managed far more effectively than if we continue to justify it, thus feeding into it. Fear is the same. We all have rational fears, the ones that seem to be part of being human, like speaking in public or going into an interview or exam. Even fear of getting sick or dying is relatively normal. But irrational fear can feed into anxiety, making it very difficult to think or function normally. Let's have a closer look at both types of fear and how to deal with them.

I once read that fear stands for 'false evidence appearing real', and this is certainly true for irrational fear, like falling off the moon. Learning to identify our fears and deciding whether they are irrational or not really does help us to separate them from the more real fears.

Fear can be generated in a number of ways, and one way is by constantly focussing on the source of the fear, but negatively, thus feeding the associated anxiety. It's natural to be a little fearful of an interview or an exam. In fact that nervousness, or even fear, triggers the adrenalin needed to give everything we have when we most need to. Making sure we have read up on the company and the job description, or studied hard, is a positive way to channel that fear. Constantly imagining that we're going to look like an idiot in the interview, or visualising the word FAIL written across our paper, is not.

The physical symptoms of fear are the same as those of anxiety, but can be more extreme; and the energy expelled living in a state of fear is huge, and very damaging, and often leads to depression.

The following method worked for me during the times I was overwhelmed by anxiety and fear. Every morning I would write a fear record based on what I was currently fearing in that moment, or my fear-based reality – and yours could include anything that you personally fear, no matter how big or small. At the end of the day I would analyse the list and keep a running total of how many fears hadn't happened and how many had. Most of the time my fears represented about three percent of my fear-based reality. Slowly it dawned on me that I was wasting a great deal of time worrying about things that never happened, which actually made me angry! But I didn't waste that anger. Instead, I harnessed it so it could be used to overcome that fear by channelling it into another emotion, like relief, even humour, that the fear hadn't come true. Combined with exercise, which for me was running at the time, I was able to decrease that morning list of fears to practically nothing...until I had nothing to write at all.

## THINGS TO TRY

In the short term, fear can be managed much the same as anxiety, by practising the breathing techniques we discussed before. Long-term fear – fear that is seriously affecting and perhaps damaging your life – needs a different approach. Here are a few ideas.

Write that list and take a good look at it. Could you stop being fearful about an exam by studying harder, or getting a study buddy to test you? Could you try the thing you are frightened of? Are any of the fears completely irrational, so that they could be crossed off the list straight away?

If you think keeping a fear record might help, try this:

For five consecutive days write down ten things you are frightened might happen. This will give you fifty things. Every morning for the next ten days check the list, and every evening take another look and see if any of the things happened. If they did, mark them; if they didn't, cross them out. At the end of the ten days add up how many fears came true and create a percentage out of one hundred. If three things from your list happened, for example, that is just six percent. Focussing on the ninety-four percent chance that your fears won't actually happen is liberating in that it might make you angry, like me, or make you laugh – I laughed too, when I stopped being angry – and allow you to channel all that wasted energy into something positive and much better for your health! Again, it might sound too simple. But the best solutions to anything often are.

# ANXIETY AND PHOBIAS

*'Your mind will answer most questions if you learn to relax and wait for the answer.'*
– William Burroughs

Phobias come under the realm of semi-irrational fear, and most have their roots in a real, though very rare, danger. Also, they are often the result of two situations.

Firstly, phobias can be the result of the natural survival signals within the brain stem, the oldest part of the survival brain, and the anxious, emotional limbic brain.

Secondly, they can be the result of collective consciousness, or learned behaviour from an early age.

A respect for heights, for example, is both a primitive prevention of injury or death, and a learned behaviour based on our parents' admonitions: 'Come away from the edge, you'll fall!' When it becomes a phobia, however, that natural survival instinct becomes a fear totally out of proportion to the risk. This is due solely to the connection between the stimulus (experiencing the fear in the conscious mind), and the emotional response that is the result of looking over the edge of the balcony: a paralysing sense of panic. This is due in part to the subconscious mind not being able to differentiate between fantasy and reality. The imagination becomes its reality – in which you plummet to your death – which causes the same psychological reaction as in reality. Before long, you are unable to even go out onto the balcony, and may not even be able to venture beyond the first floor of a building, cross a bridge, walk along a cliff...

There are so many phobias – and the list seems to grow with each passing year – but we are born with only two inbuilt fears[1] (which can develop into phobias): loud noises and falling. All the rest are learned. In the exercise below I will take two methods of treating phobias: the fast phobia cure, and the systematic desensitisation technique. In both cases

---

[1] Based on discussions by John Grinder and Richard Bandler, the founders of NLP (neuro-linguistic programming).

we will use the more common phobia of the fear of heights.

## THINGS TO TRY

### The Fast Phobia Cure

The fast phobia cure (FPC) is a rapid method of curing a phobia by using the imagination to disassociate the visual emotional tie that links a phobia to an extreme emotional reaction. There are a couple of methods used for this, but I have chosen the one that I am most familiar with. FPC is best done with a therapist who has experience in the technique, and you absolutely must want to get rid of the phobia as it is quite an intense experience.

FPC involves imagining sitting in a cinema, in a really comfy seat, and viewing a film of your phobia. But the key difference is, you separate out from yourself, as it were, in order to watch yourself watching the film of your phobia from another really comfy seat up in the gallery. (Some people opt to watch themselves from above, as if on the ceiling.) Whilst you're watching you watching the film, a favourite piece of music you've chosen is played. Either side of the film is a safe place on the screen, sometimes showing the phobia itself faded out to almost invisible, which you can focus on whilst listening to your favourite music.

At your request, the short, fast film of your phobia is played – in this case, driving across a high suspension bridge where ordinarily you would start shaking, sweating and panicking, and possibly not be able to drive at all. Whilst listening to the music, and to begin the process of disassociation from the phobia, you focus on the safe areas of the screen whilst the fast film of your phobia is played on a loop in the middle. Naturally, your eyes will keep going to the film of the phobia, creating the same symptoms as if you were actually on the bridge; but, equally, your eyes will move to the safe parts of the screen, where the symptoms begin to subside as you listen to your favourite music and even sing along if you choose.

It is quite complicated to do FPC justice in words, but it works. The combination of the 'safe spaces' that filter through to your subconscious, and the music playing, reprograms the brain to dissociate from the phobia about heights. As stated before, the brain is an incredible organ, but it believes what it is told. And you have just told it through FPC that it no longer needs to fear heights to the extent that you are immobilised and unable to function. Interestingly, the natural instinctive respect for heights remains.

**Systematic Desensitisation**

Systemic desensitisation (SD) is a very effective way of treating many phobias that interfere with life in some way. Being phobic about the red-breasted Amazon bull frog is unlikely to cause you that much trouble; but being unable to visit your daughter because she lives on the fifth floor of an apartment block will.

With SD, you will be asked to stand on a step about fifty millimetres high whilst imagining something that really relaxes you, like a sunset or a favourite place. It's really important to do this and breathe deeply and slowly as you do. Once you are comfortable standing on this step, the height is increased in increments whilst still thinking about your chosen thing and breathing deeply into the abdomen. It's amazing how quickly you will become accustomed to the height of the step, and then it is time to move outside.

The same process is applied outside, imagining the sunset or favourite place and breathing deeply as you perhaps walk with your therapist over a low bridge over the canal, or up to the second floor of an apartment block. Initially you may still get anxious, and not be able to look over the edge at the water or out of the window, but with commitment and practice you will. A good therapist will talk softly and encouragingly if you choose, maybe even take you by the arm if that's the reassurance you need, and soon you will be achieving greater and greater heights, quite literally. Not long after that you will be ringing the doorbell to your daughter's apartment, and your debilitating fear of heights will have become the primal respect we all have and not the thing that has you in a panic and running for home.

### Neuro-Linguistic Programming

NLP is the practice of using conscience language to change thoughts and behaviour, and works in a similar way to using affirmations that feed back to the subconscious brain. Some say that NLP is inconsistent with current neurological theory, but it is still a useful technique in reprogramming the brain through language.

# THE BRAIN-GUT PARADOX

*'Let food be thy medicine,*
*and medicine be thy food.'*

– Hippocrates

In the past psychologists thought that anxiety alone caused physical symptoms, especially in the intestinal system. Yet recent research has found a strange paradox. The gut itself, if unhealthy, will cause the brain to go wrong, inducing anxiety and depression. Further research has shown that the neurotransmitter serotonin (the brain's happy chemical) and dopamine (the brain's excitement and arousal chemical) are produced from substances originating in the gut. In short, the intestines and stomach seem to have their own brain, and they communicate with the brain in our heads via the vagus nervous system.

The largest cause of an unhealthy gut is connected to what we put into it, and here I will need to make a disclaimer. I am not a dietician. My advice is generalised and based on research and personal experience. It is essential you have a personal check up with your GP or a nutritionist if you think you have any intolerances, deficiencies or allergies.

The gut consists of bacteria, viruses, fungi and various other cells existing in their trillions which all work together to keep us healthy. Our unhealthy modern diet of fast or convenience food has caused the gut's balance to get out of harmony, creating conditions like depression, fatigue and a fogginess of the brain. The research is still in progress, but changing your diet might go a long way to coping with anxiety. A dysfunctional gut causes many physical symptoms like bloating, IBS, flatulence, stomach cramps, reflux, diarrhoea, constipation, belching, nausea, fatigue, colitis, and Crohn's disease. But it is also responsible for many psychological issues like anxiety and depression. By changing our diet we give our gut the best chance to react differently to the stresses of daily life which cause our anxious state.

Take a close and honest look at your diet. How much of it is good, natural food and how much is made up of fatty, sugary, or processed food? How much caffeine, alcohol or sugary drinks do you consume in a day? Do you smoke? Cigarettes and e-cigarettes, far from being ‘calming’, contain *dozens* of toxic chemicals that *trigger* anxiety not soothe it.

If you think you have a food intolerance or allergy please don’t ignore it and continue to eat the foods that upset your stomach. Seek advice and adjust your diet accordingly. A blood test can identify intolerances, allergies or deficiencies, which makes it much easier to feed your gut what it needs and avoid what makes it physically ill and, by extension, can make anxiety and depression so much worse.

If any deficiencies show up in your blood test, follow the advice of your GP or nutritionist and top up on the vitamins and minerals you are low on.

## THINGS TO TRY

Listen to the advice you have been given and listen to your body. Your gut will be trying to communicate with you through both physical and psychological symptoms. Don’t feed it the food that makes it unwell and triggers anxiety; rather, eat good brain food like oily fish, nuts, fruit and seeds, and good gut food like pro-biotic yogurts and certain fermented foods like sauerkraut, miso and sourdough. Keep a diary of what you eat and when, and how you feel afterwards.

This is a very simple thing, but it helps us to make the connection between our gut's health and our brain's health.

# DIAGNOSTIC LABELLING AND SECONDARY GAIN

*'People become attached to their burdens sometimes more than their burdens are attached to them.'*

– George Bernard Shaw

Anxiety and mental disorders are analysed on a spectrum in modern society which determine the diagnosis. There are advantages and disadvantages to diagnostic labelling, however, and this is what we'll now look at.

When people have a traumatic experience, like a car crash or the loss of someone they love, they might develop severe anxiety for the first time in their lives and not know what is happening to them. If this is unchecked it could go on to become full-blown depression, with distressing outcomes like panic attacks and unexplained aggression. It is therefore vital to speak to a professional about the original experience, and the resultant changes in how we feel, in order to work through both and hopefully process what has happened. At times like this a diagnostic label may not be required as the person can, with time and help, recover from both the experience and the effect it had on them.

Irrational anxiety, which we talked about earlier, can be a sign of depression, however, where people get a thought in their head which becomes an obsession. A client of mine became convinced he had killed someone in his car after driving past a man opening his car boot. The more he thought about this man the more convinced he was that he had killed him when he had driven past. There was absolutely no evidence to suggest the man was dead – there were no local news reports of a hit and run – but his guilt and fear consumed him. Some might have dismissed this man as a nutter and said it was obvious he hadn't killed anyone, so why was he in such a state? I gently suggested that he might be suffering from a depressive illness, and might benefit from a professional diagnosis, which he was willing to do. Interestingly, once he had been diagnosed he was able to dissociate his obsession with having killed this man from the rest of his identity as an otherwise kind and lovely son, husband and father. In this case, having a diagnostic 'label' was a huge advantage, and after several sessions with me and some mild medication he began to recover.

Labels can also work against recovery. In psychology there is a state called 'secondary gain', where some people will hold on to their anxiety or depression as they gain something from it that is lacking in their life. There are numerous reports of psychological dependency on a diagnosis – in this case a person's mental illness – to obtain sympathy, support and recognition. In this case, a label can serve to feed the situation, which is not helpful.

It is also the case that we may position ourselves almost as a vulnerable child, and adopt a helplessness that means we get the attention we need. There is lots of research on this, which we won't go into here, but learning to reframe our experiences from an adult perspective will help us deal with the symptoms of that experience as an adult, not a child. Children do not have the capacity to process life the way adults do, which is why we must guide them and support them. But we must also be our own adult. This is very important in learning to be responsible for our diagnosis and using the information to feed our recovery not our helplessness.

We must also be very honest when looking at our anxiety. Only we know the answer to whether we are perhaps using it to get sympathy and support. It's a tough question to ask ourselves, but ask it we must, and be willing to accept the answer.

Alternatively, we might be masking our anxiety because we don't want attention or sympathy, which can be just as damaging long term. In either case, honesty when considering these sensitive issues is the first step to learning to manage them.

## THINGS TO TRY

It might be good to go back to the chapter on the three types of anxiety and try to identify which type you might have. Further to this, think deeply about what might have caused the anxiety. Is something from childhood, or the more recent past? These two things are crucial steps in learning to manage your anxiety and preventing it from becoming something more serious, like depression.

Choose someone you trust and talk to them, or go to a professional and explain what is happening. The next step to recovery is accepting we are anxious and listening to advice. If we are diagnosed, then view the diagnosis as the next point of acceptance and recovery not as a thing to be ashamed of.

There are all sorts of steps we can then take, many of which we will go on to discuss.

# MANAGING A DIAGNOSIS

*'You don't have to see the whole staircase,*
*just the first step.'*
– Dr Martin Luther King

A formal diagnosis about our anxiety from a doctor or therapist can be the crucial step to learning to manage it. But how do we know when our anxiety requires intervention?

As we have discussed, natural anxiety is triggered by a brain concerned with coping with perceived threats in our lives. When the threat or risk has passed, the anxiety usually passes too. When it doesn't, and persists to the point where it is affecting our lives, then we must take action. A diagnosis can help us decide what action to take, and there are three main steps we can expect.

Firstly, there will be a discussion about how we are feeling, and what we are anxious about.

Secondly, the cause and history of our anxiety will be talked about. Has something recent triggered it, or do we think it's because of something that happened a long time ago? Is it continuous, or does it come and go? Is it worse in the morning, and where on a scale of one to ten can you place it at any particular time?

Thirdly, what are the physical signs and symptoms? Are you breathless, sweating, suffering from a dry mouth or an increased heartrate? Are you feeling nauseous, shaky or panicky? Do you notice muscle tension or repetitive back ache? Have you problems with digestion or abdominal pain?

When a diagnosis is made, don't panic as it will cause more anxiety! Listen carefully to your GP or other professional and welcome their advice. They want to help, and listening is your way of helping yourself.

## THINGS TO TRY

Try keeping a diary of the whole experience, from your first steps of seeking help and onwards through the weeks and months as you progress.

Record the triggers and symptoms, and when you feel worse and when you feel better. Keep a record of any physical responses, like any aches or pains, how frequently you need to use the bathroom, and how well (or not) you are sleeping. The more detail the better.

Write down what you are anxious about, no matter how big or small. If you are worrying about the symptoms themselves, write that down too.

Note down any changes in diet and how that affects you both mentally and physically. Be really specific about what you are eating and drinking and notice any patterns, like feeling worse after eating junk food, but better after enjoying a home-cooked meal. A friend of mine who suffered from depression and anxiety for years made the connection that when her blood sugar was low her symptoms were worse. Grazing on small, healthy snacks throughout the day really helped to stabilise her blood sugar and her symptoms.

Any action you take to help yourself feel better will work hand in hand with any advice you may be given. Take your diary with you when you visit your GP or counsellor and show them the links and patterns you have noticed. This will help them to understand your lifestyle and plan your treatment, and will help you to manage your diagnosis and your recovery.

# EPIGENETIC AND INHERITED ANXIETY

*'Act the way you want to feel.'*
– Gretchen Rubin

There is a great deal of interest as to whether anxiety is part nurture or nature, and if a gene might be responsible for memorising a trauma and passing it down through generations. Research looks at early years, and how anxiety might be etched into the psyche.

In terms of nurture, an over-protective mother, or a mother obsessed with cleanliness, is an example of learned anxiety, which can teach the child from a very early age that the world is not a safe place, or a place riddled with germs that will kill it. Abuse, whether sexual, physical or psychological, will create early trauma and deep anxiety, as will the emotional neglect of a mother who repeatedly dismisses or ignores her child's needs.

When it comes to nature, do the anxieties of great-grandparents, grandparents and parents who lived through two world wars filter down through generations of offspring, creating children more prone to PTSD (post-traumatic stress disorder), for example? We are, without doubt, the product of our genetic makeup, so is trauma passed on to our children and their children through the genes? Nobody really knows for sure. It could be that we don't inherit our ancestors' experiences directly, as we weren't there, but we inherit the echo of the experiences in terms of their reactions and ability to process and cope. This is very interesting, as to inherit the echoes of a negative experience might stop future generations repeating it...once we realise what it is and how to deal effectively with it.

Traumatic stress is a huge subject and I cannot do it justice in this book. What I will say is that early intervention is essential. Many of the shell-shocked troops of the world's wars would have had a much better chance of recovery had they been acknowledged and treated instead of being labelled as 'weak'. But whether we inherit or not, if we suspect we might be suffering from traumatic stress we must get help.

Almost all of the suggestions in this book, from individual to group therapy, to meditation and exercise, are all steps we can take to look anxiety in the face and say, 'I acknowledge you, and now I'm going to do something to help us both.'

## THINGS TO TRY

Sometimes it's helpful to tune into anxiety as the sensation that appears in the body because of it. In other words, change it from a mental thing to a physical thing. Where do you experience the anxiety? Is it in the head or gut? How big is it? What does it look like? Does it have colour? Does it have a sound, and how loud is it? If you could touch it what would it feel like?

Once you have an image of your anxiety, decide what you could do to make it smaller, quieter, softer. Can you change its colour from perhaps a bright, glaring red to a softer pink? If you visualised a blaring, horrible siren could you turn the volume down? If it was a large ball of pain, could you let some of the air out so it shrinks? These methods are used in certain branches of psychology, and are highly effective in retraining the way the brain 'sees' anxiety.

Another technique is to look at your posture. How do you stand, walk and sit? Consciously changing your stance when sitting to upright with your shoulders back instead of slumped, or walking tall rather than shuffling, feeds straight back to your subconscious that things are okay. Try it. it really does change the way you feel.

# OBSESSIVE COMPULSIVE DISORDER

*'You don't have to control your thoughts, you just have to stop letting them control you.'*

– Dan Millman

An important thing to remember about OCD is that it is actually two different things. The obsessional element of the disorder is a thinking process, and the first part. This is sometimes referred to as 'rumination disorder', where obsessional thoughts are thoughts that continually recur, over and over again. One of the characteristics of obsessional thinking is that they cannot be rationalised away. The obsessive behaviour itself is the second part.

Obsessive compulsive disorder is a behaviour triggered by an obsession, perhaps personal safety, which has the added element of becoming habitual. When treating obsessive thoughts, it is vitally important to treat the habitual aspect of the compulsion at the same time. A typical example is demonstrated by the constant checking of a door to see if it is locked. I had a client who would check the front door forty or fifty times before he went to bed, before being satisfied it was locked. When the compulsive part of his OCD was bad this would increase to checking the door forty or fifty times, every twenty minutes, completely disrupting his sleep and making his life unbearable.

Traditional psychology might suggest that the behaviour is a result of a belief system which has to change first, before the behaviour can change; but I found that treating the behaviour first has the effect of reducing the obsessive thoughts, and reducing the obsessive thoughts reduces the obsessive behaviour.

The relationship between the thought and the behaviour runs deep, and can involve all sorts of embellishments: If I don't check the door, it might still be open, and someone will get into the house and they will steal our stuff, and they will wreck the place, and the insurance won't pay up because the door was unlocked, and my partner will have a breakdown, and, and, and...

It may be said that by helping the client to stop checking the door, they will understand that everything is well, so their fears will diminish. But I strongly believe the solution is to treat both simultaneously. There is also the matter of secondary gain, where checking the door is a learned comfort that the client needs to get through the day. This must also be considered.

It's important if suffering from OCD to examine where the initial fear came from. In the above case, the client had a friend whose flat had been broken into and it triggered a panic in him that very quickly took hold. He was also fully aware that it was irrational, and felt ashamed that he couldn't control his OCD. He found comfort too in checking the door, and would enjoy momentary relief from the fear, until it came around again, and again.

## THINGS TO TRY

There are two fundamental approaches in treating OCD. The first is to work on reducing the issue systematically. By this I mean, try checking the door thirty-nine times, then thirty-eight, and so on. This works because it is a progressive way of reducing the habitual behaviour by putting you in control. It's amazing how this actually works, until checking the door once or even twice, like most of naturally do, becomes the norm.

The second approach is what's called 'exposure response prevention'. This involves doing the complete opposite to what you are obsessed about. In this example, it would mean leaving the door unlocked and asking someone else to check it, whilst repeating to yourself 'I'm comfortable leaving my door open and trusting so-and-so to lock it for me,' or even 'I'm looking forward to going out later and leaving so-and-so to lock the door for me.' This is called 'paradoxical intention', or stating the direct opposite to what your mind would normally scream at you. Another example is, 'I can't sleep, so I will stay awake.' If you've ever tried this, you'll know how quickly you fall asleep!

It may seem odd, but behaving in a way opposite to your obsession means you take control of it, and quickly diminish it.

# TRADITIONAL VERSUS ALTERNATIVE THERAPY

*'Difficult roads often lead to beautiful destinations.'*
– Zig Ziglar

There are many types of therapist who use different techniques to help with anxiety, both traditional and alternative. In essence, any cognitive intervention that is part of statutory psychiatry practice can be classed as therapy, and although it may seem like a hard thing to begin, the results are definitely worth aiming for. I won't go into all the types of therapy, as there are too many, but I'll cover a few key ones here.

A traditional counsellor is trained to listen in a very special way. The best counsellors will encourage you to talk, gently guiding your thoughts in the direction of a successful outcome. For many anxious individuals this is a very beneficial technique as it brings the deeper reasons for the anxiety to the surface where we are able to see them, perhaps for the first time, as symptoms that can be managed and eventually conquered.

Psychotherapists have been trained in various disciplines and often use CBT, or cognitive behavioural therapy, to identify negative cognitions – or distorted thoughts and their associated habits – and replace them with positive affirmations and thinking. Cognitive therapy is 'present focused' and doesn't always rely on digging up past traumas to effect a cure. In this respect it is highly effective for those who don't wish to dwell on the past but instead focus on making the present, and consequently the future, a calmer, happier place where anxiety can be managed as and when it arises.

If you are more of a social person, group counselling can be very comforting because we realise we are not alone, particularly if our anxiety is because of a very specific thing, like abuse or rape. People who have been through a particular trauma can get great help from others who have had a similar experience. Group therapy can also involve role play between the group members present, which helps develop strong relationships within the group and acts as a support mechanism. Groups are not for everyone, however, as some of us are more private, so if you join a group but do not feel comfortable do not cause yourself more anxiety by staying.

Mindfulness, which many consider 'alternative' and yet has been around for thousands of years through meditation, follows a similar approach in encouraging us to be in the moment. It does this through using body awareness and breathing, which can only happen in the present moment: you can't be aware of your body and breath in the past as it has passed; and you can't be aware in the future as it hasn't arrived yet. Because so much of our anxiety is based on past events, or on events in the future that may or may not happen, mindfulness is a gentle, very effective way to manage anxiety.

Other 'alternative' or 'complimentary' therapies that have been around for thousands of years are herbal remedies, acupuncture and reflexology, for instance. Many challenge these therapies on the basis that they lack the scientific rigour of traditional interventions, but anybody who has felt the benefit of an hour of reflexology or a session of acupuncture would challenge that view. I worked closely with several complimentary therapists when I had my practice, with the GP's blessing, and saw vast improvements in both the mental and physical health of my clients.

The most important thing here is to do what works for you. You will know when something feels right as you will feel your anxiety ease.

## THINGS TO TRY

When you make the decision to get professional help from a therapist do some research first or get your GP to recommend someone. Good therapists will have proper qualifications and be on the national register. Make sure you feel absolutely comfortable with your therapist, or you will not be able to open up to them. Don't develop a false sense of loyalty and stay with a therapist because you feel you ought to, which will cause more anxiety. Try different ones until you 'click' with someone, and stay open to their suggestions and guidance.

The same is true with group therapy. Try different groups until you feel comfortable and able to talk to the people around you. The bonds that are forged in group therapy are incredibly healing, but don't expect to get along with everybody. You just need to feel safe and comfortable.

Mindfulness practice can be done alone or in groups, and in online groups. Do some reading on the subject and try different methods, as there are lots. You will know when you have found the right practice or group for you as you will naturally relax.

Maybe book yourself a reflexology session, which works by stimulating the parts of the body directly linked to points in your feet. Most people find it a deeply relaxing therapy which benefits the entire body, as it eases tension and promotes healing.

# HYPNOSIS

*'The best weapon against stress is our ability to choose one thought over another.'*

– William James

What is hypnosis? In essence it is a means of bypassing the mind's constant conscious chatter and going straight to the subconscious. There are three states of hypnosis: **suggestion, the alpha state** and **somnambulism.**

Hypnosis is a very powerful way of reframing negative thinking by appealing directly to the subconscious mind. (I used hypnosis within my practice with great effect.) There is a great deal of rubbish and false belief surrounding hypnosis, however, usually instigated by dreadful stage shows that seem to take delight in humiliating individuals for profit, and the cynics who do not believe hypnosis works. Let's have a look at the three states in more detail.

**Suggestion** does not involve any form of trance and can actually be achieved alone, and is best achieved by repetition through affirmations. The basic idea is to make a statement to yourself over and over again that is the opposite to your anxiety, without attempting to emotionalise it. For instance, if using public transport makes you anxious and your mind keeps saying, 'I hate getting the train to work; I hate trains,' replace this with 'I love the fact I can watch the countryside go by when I'm on the train,' or 'Getting the train to work gives me a chance to read another chapter of my book.' Over time your subconscious will override the anxiety relating to a particular event, or imagined event, by replacing it with something more positive.

**The alpha state** does involve a mild form of trance, and is similar to the day-dream state in the present, or the period just before you go to sleep and just as you wake up. This state can be explored with a qualified hypnotherapist using a process of guided imagery, allowing you to imagine a scene that relaxes the chatter of the conscious mind. There is in fact a very close link between the alpha state and the meditative state, which has excellent short- and long-term benefits for an overly busy and anxious mind. This can be achieved with a hypnotherapist, but it can also be a practice to try alone through learning to still the mind's chatter through meditation. A hypnotherapist will guide you through a series of questions in this state, whereby you can access the deeper sources of anxiety, like past hurts and traumas, and reprogram the beliefs that those events created.

**Somnambulism** is a deeper state of hypnosis, similar to the sleepwalker's mind. This can be induced using an ideomotor response, a reflex muscle action from the unconscious mind that is then deepened by progressive induction techniques like descending stairs or total body relaxation. I found that where hypnosis was helpful, most clients did not need the deeper state of somnambulism. The brain is a most remarkable organ, and suggestion and the alpha state were almost always sufficient to achieve the results required.

If you decide to try hypnotherapy, make sure the therapist is qualified and registered. Hypnotherapy is a perfectly safe technique in the hands of a professional, and alongside honest discussions with a counsellor or psychotherapist can target anxiety where it takes root: deep in the subconscious brain.

## THINGS TO TRY

If your anxiety is crippling, you may well benefit from a few sessions of hypnotherapy to get to that deep part of the brain and reprogram it. Don't believe the rubbish written about hypnotherapy and find a therapist you are relaxed with. Trust them to do the job they have trained long and hard to do.

The two states of mind most commonly achieved through hypnosis – suggestion and the alpha state – can be practised at home too through meditation, which we will discuss in the next chapter.

# MEDITATION

*'Peace is the result of retraining your mind*
*to process life as it is*
*rather than as you think it should be.'*

– Wayne Dyer

Meditation is immensely powerful for focussing on the present, and thus allowing the past and the future to stay where they belong. Despite all of our stories of the past, and our imaginings of the future, life actually only happens in the present moment, and focussing on this is incredibly calming when we are anxious. Going quiet, concentrating on our breathing and noticing each sensation in our body – where we are tense or in pain, for instance, and spending a few moments with that tension or pain – instantly slows the heartrate and allows us to gather ourselves, as it were. This can be done wherever you are. And if you are struggling to sleep, this practice will calm your mind and body. If you struggle to concentrate with this, there are lots of short and long sleep meditations on YouTube. Yoga Nidra meditations are particularly effective.

But meditation can also be used to access the deeper subconscious beliefs we have harboured which may still be causing us anxiety. In the meditative state, it is always interesting what 'comes up', and by noticing we are often able to go straight to the original cause of the anxiety, and the symptoms, and create a state of acceptance and healing. No harm will ever come from practicing meditation. It is well documented how our mental and physical health benefits from just a few minutes a day spent calming our chattering, anxious mind.

## THINGS TO TRY

This is a short meditation I used many times to calm my anxiety. It is now part of my daily routine.

Choose a time and find a place where you will not be disturbed. Turn off your phone and all other devices.

Sit comfortably and take a couple of deep breaths. If it helps you to relax play quiet, soothing music in the background. But make sure it's not music that you will start noticing for any particular reason, like a triggered memory.

As you breathe deeply, focus on your feet. Let them relax. Notice each toe, and your ankles, and let them relax too.

Now focus on your lower legs, and then your thighs, and imagine them getting heavier as they relax into the chair.

Focus on your abdomen. Let it go heavy too. Do the same for your chest and your arms and shoulders. Let them all relax until they feel heavy. Feel the chair against your back, and your arms by your sides. Sink deeper into the relaxation.

Finally, let your neck and face relax. Imagine the muscles going soft under your skin. Feel the weight of your head. Release the tension around your eyes. Keep your head up, but soft, feeling the whole body sink into the chair.

Now your body is relaxed, go to a place in your mind that you love. We all have a special place, like a park or a quiet beach or a garden. What do you notice? What can you hear and smell? Maybe the sun is on your face, or a slight breeze is in the trees, or the waves are breaking on the sand. How do you feel? Are you safe and content? Feel that safety and contentment. *Really* feel it and enjoy it. Notice the sensations, like the air on your skin or the sand under your feet. Sink into it. All of it.

When you are ready, slowly bring your attention back to the weight of your body in the chair, and the sounds and sensations in the present. Notice your breath again. Focus on how it moves in and out of your body.

When you are ready, stretch your hands and arms, feet and legs and back. Hunch your shoulders and relax them. Move your head from side to side. Wake everything up. You are ready to begin the next part of your day.

This simple practice is deeply calming for the mind and the body. It allows for a pause in our hectic lives, and helps us to accept and even embrace the 'what is' of life and be at peace with it. There are no rules about when or for how long, but try to practice this as often as you can.

# EXERCISE

*'Take care of your body. It's the only place you have to live.'*

– Jim Rohn

All mental health care workers agree that exercise is one of the most effective ways of managing stress, anxiety and worry. This is because when you exercise, you burn off much of the adrenalin released in the fight, flight or freeze situation. Exercise also generates chemicals in the body called endorphins which make you feel good by eliminating the feelings associated with anxiety. Studies show that aerobic exercise is as good as practising abdominal breathing when it comes to reducing panic attacks. We are all in a different physical state, age and situation, and how and when we exercise differs from person to person. But the key thing is: Find a form of exercise you enjoy, and fits your age and lifestyle, and do it!

However, despite the fact that most people know that exercise is good for them and will make them feel better, many still decide not to. There are three main reasons for this.

Firstly, a reluctance to exercise may be because of childhood trauma. Maybe you had a negative experience at school because exercise involved being bullied by much fitter children, or you hated your body because it was too fat or too thin, or you were simply rubbish at sports and always felt like you made a fool of yourself.

Secondly, some people think that exercise will actually do them harm. This belief might be because of an injury or an illness that weakened you, and left you trapped in a subconscious mindset that wants to protect you from further injury. This happened to a friend of mine after knee surgery. She had become so used to protecting the original injury that after surgery she became fearful of the physio required to return her to full physical health.

Finally, perhaps you don't exercise because you find it boring or too much effort. All that moving about and sweating...

If any of the above apply, have a look at the following.

**THINGS TO TRY**

The **FITT – frequency, intensity, time** and **type – principle** takes into consideration almost every type of aerobic (increases heartrate) and anaerobic (improves muscle function) exercise there is. There are three important things to consider before you begin.

Firstly, before you start any new exercise, if you have concerns about your physical health book a check-up with your GP to ensure that you are safe to exercise.

Secondly, make sure you have easy, comfortable clothes to wear and the appropriate footwear.

Thirdly, choose an exercise that you enjoy and that will be relatively effortless to begin. Don't decide to start swimming if you live miles from a public pool and hate cold (ish) water! And don't choose running if you wrecked your knees playing rugby at school! You get the idea...

Once you've had your check-up, found some suitable clothes, and picked a form of exercise you enjoy, you can employ the FITT principle, which means applying one improvement element at a time.

**F for frequency.** You increase the number of times you exercise each week.

**I for intensity.** You increase how hard you exercise at each visit.

**T for time**. You increase the time you exercise on each visit.

**T for type.** You expand the type of exercise you try.

By increasing one element at a time, in rotation, your overall fitness will improve gradually, reducing the chance of injury and loss of motivation.

I know we mentioned a dislike of swimming, but swimming is a great overall exercise. Your body weight is supported, and it rarely causes muscle strain if lengths and speed are increased in implements as per the FITT principle.

Walking is excellent exercise, but make sure you have proper, supportive boots or trainers. Again, the distance and speed can be increased incrementally, and the extra benefits for anxiety management are being in the fresh air and amongst nature, which is calming and restorative.

Dancing can be done in your living room or as part of a dance class, and is a fun and highly social form of exercise. It releases lots of endorphins, and focusses the brain as you learn the steps.

Yoga is becoming more and more popular as people notice the deeply calming effects of the breathing, the movements and the poses. It is known to boost the immune system, lower blood pressure and create an almost meditative state that is perfect for managing anxiety. The body becomes strong and supple, and the chattering mind is hushed.

These are just a few of dozens of types of exercise you could try. And it's true that once you start you want to do more because of the way the body and brain responds to movement: It makes it feel good, so it wants more.

If you still find you get a bit bored, or can't quieten your busy mind, maybe listen to audio books or podcasts or some of your favourite music. In short, try anything that gets you off the sofa, out of your mind and into your body, where the healing of anxiety can begin.

# NATURE AND ANIMALS

*'Look deep into nature,
and then you will understand everything better.'*
– Albert Einstein

The natural world is one of the most therapeutic ways of dealing with anxiety, and it is all around us. Even if you live in the city, like I do, you don't usually have to walk very far to be near trees and plants. Even a pot plant on a windowsill or on your desk can have a very calming effect when you focus on it for a few moments.

Nature does not judge or care about what we look like, it is just there, being itself. It doesn't worry that it hasn't rained for ages, or it has rained too much, or about what might happen if it never rained again... Nature isn't anxious.

Walking through a park or in the woods we sense an order and deep calm that can be lacking as anxious human beings. It reminds us that there is a huge, incredible universe around us, also just being itself.

This may seem overwhelming to think about at first, until we compare it to our own remarkable bodies, which also just get on with being themselves by breathing and digesting food and healing injuries. Nature has a built-in rhythm that corresponds to our own and noticing this has a very quietening effect on our chattering minds. There are also much richer levels of oxygen near trees as they expel oxygen into the atmosphere, which helps to clear the brain. It is important to remember that we are part of nature, not separate from it, and we all share a harmonic rhythm of life which is deeply healing.

The same is true of animals, as anybody who has a dog or a cat will tell you. The loyalty and love they have for us, running up to greet us when we get home and sitting at our feet or curled up on our laps, instantly makes us smile and relax. People who work with animals, or volunteer at animal sanctuaries, always speak about how calming it is to be with them, caring for them and feeling them relax as they are stroked. Some hospitals use pet therapy to calm anxious or sick patients, and the results are astonishing in terms of both mental and physical recovery.

If you can't have a pet for any reason – perhaps your landlord won't allow it – try to spend some of your spare time around animals, like a friend's dog, for example. Lots of people offer dog-walking services (which is excellent exercise!), or cat-sitting whilst their owner is away. Maybe this would be a way for you to get closer to animals?

## THINGS TO TRY

Try to spend some time in nature every day, even just for a few minutes. If you are lucky enough to live near the sea, go down to the shore and breathe the oxygen-rich air deep into your lungs.

Keep plants in your house or office. Even the act of caring for a plant, watering and feeding it, has a calming effect. And spending a few moments observing how it quietly goes about its life of being a plant without any stress is surprisingly soothing.

If you can't keep a pet at home, offer to walk your friend's dog while they're at work, or look after their cat when they're away. Maybe even volunteer at an animal sanctuary. The loyalty and love animals have for us takes us out of our own anxious heads and into theirs. Taking in a rescue dog or cat is also deeply calming, and very often the healing happens together as you get to know each other.

# HUMOUR

*'We laugh for a reason,*
*so always find a reason to laugh.'*

– K L Miller

It is a well-known phrase that 'laughter is the best medicine'. I would also like to suggest that humour has a massive influence on reducing anxiety. I believe we developed a sense of humour specifically to override the negative effects of stress, and to share the very human activity of a good old laugh with friends. One of the first things we do is teach our babies to smile and laugh. Even certain animals seem to have a sense of humour, deliberately playing around and even appearing to laugh at themselves. Yes, humour is a survival technique that, if lacking, makes life feel very empty.

When we are anxious and depressed laughing is the last thing we feel like doing, or can even imagine ourselves doing, so how can we learn to laugh more, and when we most need it?

Laughing, like exercise, releases endorphins in the brain, and what we find funny can be both a very individual and collective thing. A friend of mine has children who will sit and laugh their socks off watching old Monty Python films with her, but her mother watches with a very puzzled look on her face...! When you find something you find funny, both alone and in company, remember it. Put the old film on, or watch some Micky Flannigan (or Woody Allen, or whoever makes you laugh loudly!) sketches on YouTube, or get someone to tell the funny story of when you all went camping and a cow walked in the tent door! Print some lines from a film that always make you laugh, or other quotes, and keep them close by. My editor has a wooden plaque next to her desk that says, 'What if the Hokey Cokey really is what it's all about?', which always makes her laugh, and which she no doubt looks at frequently when editing my books...

In short, just laugh. It doesn't matter what about. Try to see the humour in every situation, even your own anxiety and behaviour. How many times did I check the door? Why on earth was I afraid of the inside of Crème Eggs? Life is crazy, and sad, and infuriating, but there is always, always something to laugh about.

## THINGS TO TRY

Write down all your favourite funny films and watch them when you're feeling particularly anxious. Even twenty minutes over lunch of something funny can release anxiety and help you get through the afternoon.

When you get together with friends or family, spend time laughing about some of the good times and funny things that you've shared together. Even that time itself can become a funny, happy memory.

Print some 'funnies' and keep them on your desk or the wall in the kitchen. Buy funny postcards and add them to the collection.

To conclude, learn to laugh at life, at yourself, at the situations and scrapes we all get into and survive. We laugh for a reason, so always find a reason to laugh.

# CONCLUSION

*'Move, but not the way fear makes you move.'*

– Rumi

This book was written from the heart by someone overwhelmed by multiple anxieties for years. I hope you've found a little comfort, and some things to try which might help you learn to manage and even conquer your own personal anxieties.

It might sound crazy, but if you are naturally an anxious person, don't try not be anxious. The effort in avoiding being anxious actually makes you more anxious! The goal really is to bring your anxiety under control by taking proactive action on a daily basis, whether through mindfulness, breathing, exercise, diet, therapy...whatever works for you. Indeed, the energy of anxiety can actually be channelled into creativity and activities that are transformative.

It is through suffering that we can become compassionate, empathetic human beings; but we don't have to suffer alone or for ever. By overcoming our anxiety, and our fears, we can really start living.

I wish you all the very best.

*Peter Bull*

# ALSO IN THE GET IN TOUCH SERIES

I have found that succinct information that gets to the roots of what we seek to learn is highly effective. The **GET IN TOUCH** series of books and audiobooks is therefore designed to be short and to the point.

**GET IN TOUCH:** With Your Public Voice

**GET IT TOUCH:** With Your Inner Wealth

**GET IN TOUCH:** With Your Slimmer Self

**GET IN TOUCH:** With Your Universe

Your feedback as a reader is always welcome, and more information on the **GET IN TOUCH** series can be found on my website:

**www.getintouchbooks.com**

*Available worldwide from Amazon*

---

Michael Terence
Publishing

www.mtp.agency

www.facebook.com/mtp.agency

@mtp_agency

Printed in Great Britain
by Amazon

72024487R00061